IMPORTANT INFORMATION:

This book is intended to be used as a reference book by qualified medical or fitness professionals. Thus, anyone using the exercises listed in this book without appropriate training in the field of fitness and exercise, or without the prior consent of a physician or therapeutic professional, may be placing themselves at risk for an injury. The exercises are provided as options, *not prescriptions*, and are therefore to be used in concert with an experienced professional's education and guidelines. VHI is not responsible or liable, directly or indirectly, for any damages whatsoever resulting in injury from the information contained in this work.

CONTENTS

Introduction

The material in this collection is designed for medical and fitness professionals who work with the strength needs of patients and clients. It is a compilation of exercise ideas and options for the lower body.

This work brings together the creativity of many experts in fitness and rehabilitation who have designed "kits" for Visual Health Information (Tacoma, WA). It is not the purpose or intent of this collection to represent each and every possible exercise option for each part of the body. Nor is it the intent to describe and define when and how to use or not use any one exercise for any particular client or athlete, especially where a therapeutic consideration is warranted. Rather, it is designed simply as a resource, a reference for those who help others get in shape, to improve function or form.

Therapists and trainers often have limited resources - either working with a minimum of gym equipment or in people's homes. Creativity is important under these circumstances. When a client's unique needs or interests confront a therapist or trainer, his understanding of biomechanics and anatomy may be challenged in ways that require him to search for options. This collection was designed and should be used to find ways to get the same results with a variety of methods.

Exercise Ideas for the Lower Body provides the trainer with over 180 exercises for the muscles and joints below the waist. For simplicity, the chapters are laid out in an orderly fashion with an attempt to minimize crossover. Due to the nature of the lower body's relation to the ground, most of the chapters are divided into what are called "open chain" and "closed chain" exercises. "Open chain" exercises are those in which the distal segment, in this case the foot, is not in contact with a nearly-immovable or immovable resistance. As such, the lower leg will move as if free in space when the knee muscles contract; or the foot will move in free space when the ankle muscles contract. "Closed chain" exercises are those in which the distal segment, the foot, is in contact with a nearly-immovable or immovable resistance. Thus, exercises on machines where the bottom of the foot presses onto a plate, even if the plate (or the seat/bench) slides, would be considered closed chain.

Finally, as in any book of this nature, a disclaimer is necessary. Thus, anyone using the exercises listed in this book without appropriate training in the field of fitness and exercise, or without the prior consent of a physician or therapeutic professional, may be placing his/her clients or him- or herself at risk for an injury. The exercises are provided as options, not prescriptions, and are therefore to be used in concert with an experienced professional's education and guidelines.

Chapter 1: Total Leg Exercises

This chapter consists of those exercises that use all the muscles of the lower body, more or less. That is, those exercises that are not constrained by the path of a machine's guide rods or levers and use the stabilizing of the hip adductors and abductors and the lower leg/ankle muscles, not just the quadriceps, hamstrings, gluteals, and gastrocnemius. These exercises are often part of the core lifts in most exercise programs, especially for athletes. They are now more recognized for their rehabilitation value since they are closed-chain exercises. In fact, with the aging population's need for power, function, and bone-development, the Total Leg exercises are being promoted at all levels of fitness and wellness.

General considerations, of muscle function are as follows:
- A. The more the knee flexes, the greater the quadriceps activation and the patellofemoral stress.
- B. The more the hip flexes, the greater the hamstrings and gluteal (especially, gluteus maximus) activation and the risk of technique and/or spinal stability failure.
- C. The narrower the stance, in a free-standing exercise, the more hip and ankle stabilization is required, hence the greater the hip abduction/adduction and gastrocnemius/tibialis anterior/peroneal activation.
- D. Spinal stability and core strength are very important during all of these lifts, especially those in free space.

Total Leg exercises use many if not all of the following muscles: Quadriceps, Hamstrings, Gluteals, Adductors, Abductors, Gastrocnemius/Soleus, Peroneals.

Body Weight - 11 exercises
Resisted - 23 exercises
Machines - 8 exercises

Wall Sit

Back against wall, slide down so knees are at 90° angle. Hold.

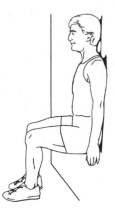

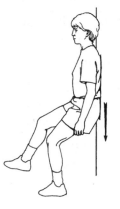

Single-Leg Quarter Squat: Quad Strength

Standing on involved leg with back against wall, slide down wall until knee is at 30-45°. Return.

Squat (Aquatic)

Bend both knees lowering body. Straighten knees and raise body.

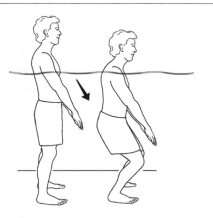

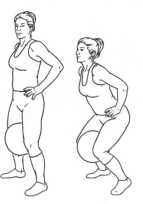

Mini Squat: with Ball Squeeze

Stand with ball between knees. Squat with head up, reaching back with buttocks as if sitting down.

Full Squat: Body Weight

Head up, back straight, feet pointed slightly out, squat until backs of thighs touch calves. Adjust arm position for balance. Keep abdominals tight and maintain weight on heels.

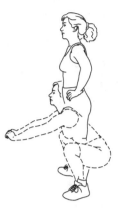

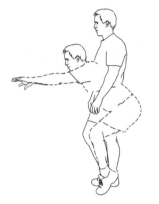

Mini Squat: 1.5 Legs

With feet shoulder width apart, raise left foot onto toes. Reach forward for balance and do a mini squat. Keep knees in line with second toe. Knees do not go past toes.

Mini Squat: Single-Leg

Stand on right foot. Reach forward for balance and do a mini squat. Keep knees in line with second toe. Knees do not go past toes. Keep knees together.

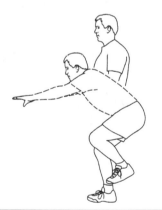

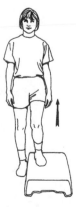

Single-Leg Step-Up: Quad Strength

With foot of involved leg on step, straighten leg. Return.

Forward Step-Up: Proprioception, Quad Strength, Timing, Coordination

Move onto step with one foot, then the other. Step back off the same way.

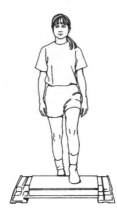

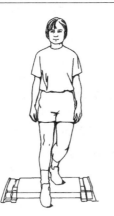

Retro Step-Up: Proprioception, Coordination, Quad Strength

Step on backwards with one foot, then the other. Step off forward the same way.

Side Step-Up: Proprioception, Quad Strength, Coordination

Step up sideways with one foot, then the other. Step off other side the same way.

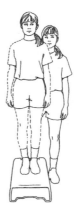

Squat Supported (Dumbbell)

Back straight, bend knees, but do not allow them past toes.

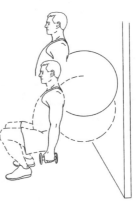

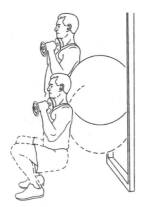

Squat Supported: Front (Dumbbell)

Back straight, dumbbells at shoulders. Bend at hips; do not allow knees past toes.

Parallel Squat (Dumbbell)

Back straight, head up, bend knees until thighs are parallel to floor. Keep abdominals tight and maintain weight on heels.

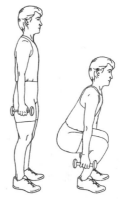

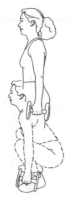

Full Squat (Dumbbell)

Head up, back straight, feet pointed slightly out, squat until backs of thighs touch calves. Keep abdominals tight and maintain weight on heels.

Back Parallel Squat (Barbell)

Back straight, head up, bend knees until
thighs are parallel to floor. Keep abdominals
tight and maintain weight on heels.

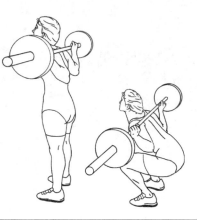

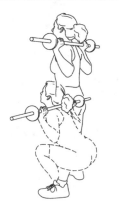

Back Full Squat (Barbell)

Head up, back straight, feet pointed slightly out,
squat until backs of thighs touch calves. Keep
abdominals tight and maintain weight on heels.

Front Full Squat (Barbell)

Bar in front, head up, back straight, feet
pointed slightly out, squat until backs
of thighs touch calves. Keep abdominals
tight and maintain weight on heels.

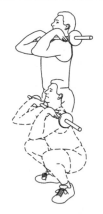

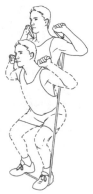

Squat

In shoulder width stance, anchor tubing
under feet. Palms forward at shoulder
height. Squat, keeping back straight.

Squat Supported: Lateral (Dumbbell)

Back straight, lean into ball. Bend at knee; do not allow knees past toes. Repeat on same side, legs switched. Repeat sequence on other side.

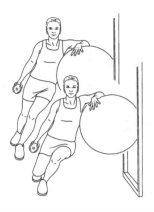

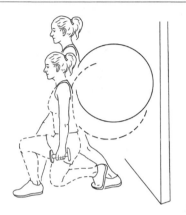

Squat-Split Supported (Dumbbell)

Back straight, bend at knee; do not allow knees past toes. Repeat with other leg forward.

Squat-Split Foot on Ball

Back straight. Do not allow knees past toes. Repeat with other leg on ball.

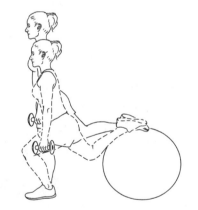

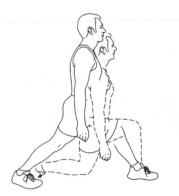

Lunge: Stationary

In wide stride, legs shoulder width apart, head up, back straight, bend both legs simultaneously until forward thigh is parallel to floor. Do all repetitions to one side. Repeat on other side.

Lunge (Dumbbell)

Legs shoulder width apart, head up, back
straight, step forward bending same leg until
thigh is parallel to floor. Alternate legs.

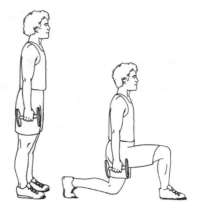

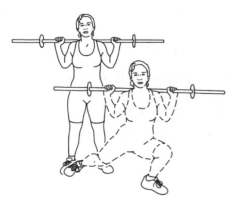

Lunge: Stationary (Barbell)

In wide stride, legs shoulder width apart, head
up, back straight, bend both legs simultaneously
until forward thigh is parallel to floor. Do all
repetitions to one side. Repeat on other side.

Lunge (Barbell)

Legs shoulder width apart, head up, back
straight, step forward bending same leg until
thigh is parallel to floor. Alternate legs.

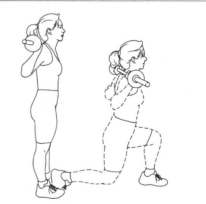

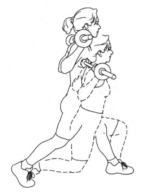

Lunge: Side (Barbell)

Head up, back straight, step forward and
to side, bending forward leg until thigh
is parallel with floor. Alternate legs.

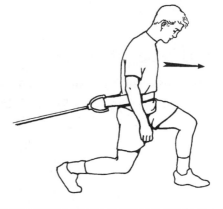

Lunge With Tubing: Quad Strength

With tubing around waist, push off with one foot and lunge forward onto the other. Return. Alternate legs. Advance with each lunge.

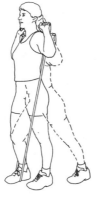

Lunge Step: Backward (Beginning)

In stride stance, anchor tubing under forward foot. Palms forward at shoulder height. Step back with other leg, keeping it straight.

Lunge Step: Backward (Advanced)

In stride stance, anchor tubing under forward foot. Palms forward at shoulder height. Step back with other leg, allowing it to flex.

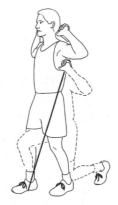

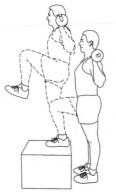

Step-Up (Barbell)

Head up, back straight, step up on box, bringing other leg up toward chest. Alternate step-up leg.

Step-Up (Dumbbell)

Head up, back straight, step up on box, bringing other leg up toward chest. Alternate step-up leg.

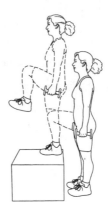

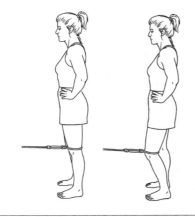

Terminal Knee Extension (Standing)

Facing anchor with left knee slightly bent and tubing just above knee, gently pull knee back straight. Do not overextend knee.

Knee Co-Contraction: Standing (Single-Leg)

Shoulder width stance, loop band just above knee and anchor behind. Loop another just below knee and anchor in front. Perform a partial squat, then straighten knee.

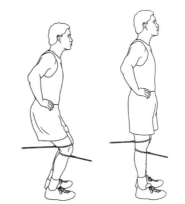

Back Full Squat (Smith Machine)

Head up, back straight, squat until backs of thighs touch calves. Keep abdominals tight and maintain weight on heels.

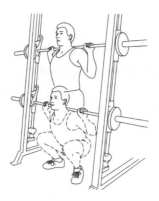

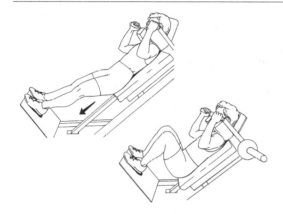

Parallel Squat (Hack Squat Machine)

Legs shoulder width apart, head up, bend knees until thighs are parallel to foot board. Keep abdominals tight and maintain weight on heels.

Parallel Squat (Power Squat Machine)

Back straight, head up, bend knees until thighs are parallel to foot board. Keep abdominals tight, maintain weight on heels.

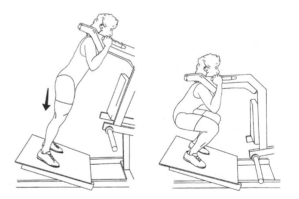

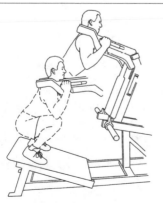

Full Squat (Power Squat Machine)

Back straight, head up, squat until backs of thighs touch calves. Keep abdominals tight and maintain weight on heels.

Full Squat (Hack Squat Machine)

Back straight, head up, squat until backs of thighs touch calves. Keep abdominals tight and maintain weight on heels.

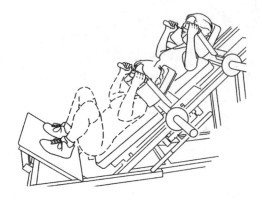

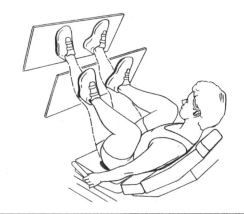

Leg Press: Incline (Machine)

Press forward until legs are just short of locked knee position.

Leg Press (Machine)

Press forward until knees are just short of locked position.

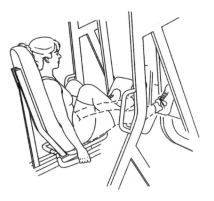

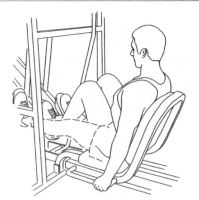

Leg Press: Single-Leg (Machine)

Press forward until knee is just short of locked position.

Chapter 2:
Quadriceps/Hip Flexors Exercises

The quadriceps, or quads, are comprised of the four muscles on the front of the thigh. They consist of the rectus femoris (the two-joint muscle that acts at the hip and the knee), vastus lateralis (on the outer aspect of the thigh), the vastus intermedius (beneath the rectus femoris), and the vastus medialis (the tear-drop shape muscle on the lower, medial aspect of the thigh). The vastus medialis is recognized as most important for proper tracking of the patella, as it pulls the patella medially as the knee extends. All four work to extend the knee; the rectus femoris also flexes the hip. The other hip flexor is the iliopsoas, a combination muscle including the iliacus, originating from the anterior lower lumbar vertebrae, and melding with the psoas, which originates from the anterior ilium, with their common insertion on the upper femur.

While all of the exercises in the Total Leg chapter also engage the quads, especially as the angle of the knee flexion increases, these were not included in this chapter because they are not specific to the quadriceps. The exercises listed here are primarily open-chain exercises that focus on the quadriceps as knee extensors and/or hip flexors.

Exercises for the quads engage most or all of the following muscles: Rectus Femoris, Vastus Lateralis, Vastus Intermedius, Vastus Medialis; Iliopsoas.

Open Chain - 19 exercises

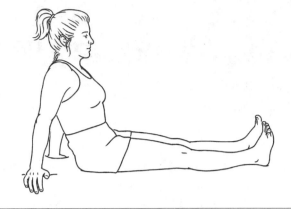

Quadriceps Set: Strengthening

Tighten muscles on top of thighs by pushing knees down into surface. Hold.

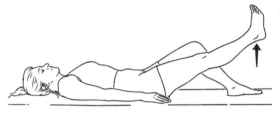

Straight Leg Raise (Phase 1): Strengthening

Tighten muscles on front of right thigh, then lift leg from surface, keeping knee locked. Hold.

Straight Leg Raise (Phase 2): Strengthening

Resting on forearms, tighten muscles on front of thigh, then lift leg from surface, keeping knee locked. Hold.

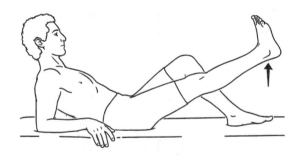

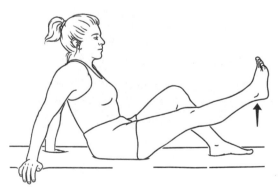

Straight Leg Raise (Phase 3): Strengthening

Resting on hands, tighten muscles on front of thigh, then lift leg from surface, keeping knee locked. Hold.

Straight Leg: with Bent Knee (Supine)

With one leg straight, other leg bent, raise straight leg. Hold.

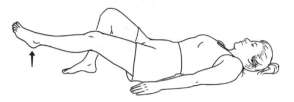

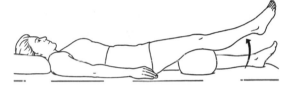

Terminal Knee Extension (Supine): Strengthening

With knee over bolster, straighten knee by tightening muscles on top of thigh. Keep bottom of knee on bolster. Hold.

Knee Flexion / Extension (Sitting): Self-Mobilization

Gently push weak leg back with other leg until a stretch is felt. Hold. Relax. Recross bent legs at ankles. Slowly straighten legs, pushing with lower leg. Hold.

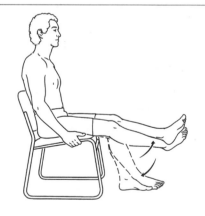

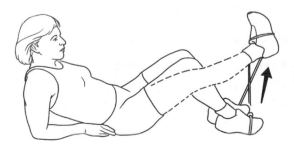

Knee Extension: Hook-Lying (Single-Leg)

Reclined sitting with arm support, tubing around feet with a twist between. Straighten one knee.

Leg Raise: Straight - Hook-Lying (Single-Leg)

Reclined sitting, one leg straight, with arm support, anchor tubing around both feet. Lift straight leg.

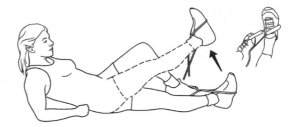

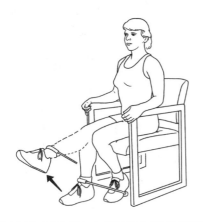

Knee Extension: Sitting (Single-Leg)

Anchor tubing under back foot. With loop around other ankle, straighten knee.

Leg Extension (Machine)

Straighten legs to locked knee position, keeping toes flexed toward knees.

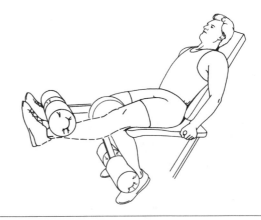

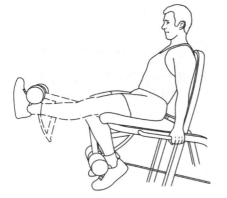

Extension: Single-Leg (Machine)

Straighten leg to locked knee position, keeping foot flexed toward knee.

Knee Extension / Flexion, Hip Flexed

Lift leg forward, bending knee. Straighten knee and lift foot, then bend knee and return to start.

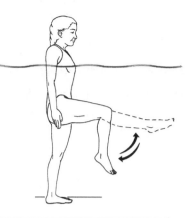

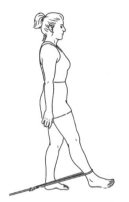

Hip Flexion – Resisted: Strengthening

With tubing around ankle, anchor behind, bring leg forward, keeping knee straight.

Hip / Glute Flexion Standing (Machine)

Leg over pad behind, bring knee forward and up as high as possible.

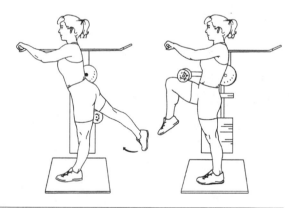

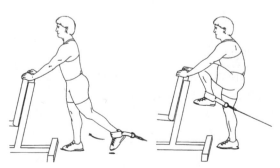

Hip / Glute Flexion Standing (Cable)

Holding support, bring knee forward and up as high as possible.

Hip Flexion: Standing (Single-Leg)

Face away from anchor in wide stride stance, tubing looped around ankle. Flex hip and knee forward.

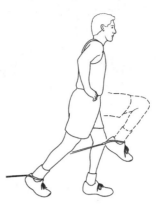

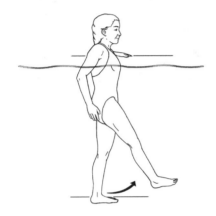

Hip Flexion, Knee Straight (Aquatic)

Lift straight leg forward and up.

Retro Stool Walk: Quad Strength

Using both legs, "walk" backward down a long hall.

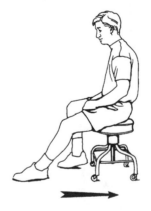

Chapter 3: Hamstrings

The hamstrings are the muscles on the posterior aspect of the thigh. They consist of the biceps femoris (a two-joint, lateral-thigh muscle that flexes the knee and extends the hip), the semitendinosus (the superficial, medial muscle), and the semimembranosus (the deeper medial muscle). The hamstrings are considered very instrumental in knee stability yet are overlooked in most exercise programs. Because of their insertions on the lateral and medial posterior tibia, they also have a rotational movement at the knee. Rarely operating as open-chain movers of the lower leg, they function primarily as closed-chain knee stabilizers and hip mobilizers. Hamstrings have been thought to hamper movement and cause low back pain. However, most experts now recognize that strong and supple hamstrings prevent injury to themselves and the low back.

While all of the exercises in the Total Leg chapter also engage the hamstrings, especially as the angle of the knee flexion increases, these were not included in this chapter because they are not specific to the hamstrings. The exercises listed here are primarily open-chain exercises that focus on the hamstrings as knee flexors and/or hip extensors.

Hamstring exercises use the following muscles: Semitendinosus, Semimembranosus, Biceps Femoris.

> **Open Chain - 19 exercises**
> **Closed Chain - 15 exercises**

Knee Flexion: Resisted (Sitting)

Sit with band under one foot and looped around ankle of supported leg. Pull unsupported leg back.

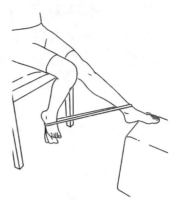

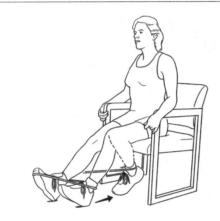

Knee Flexion: Sitting (Single-Leg)

Legs extended, anchor loop around one foot. Put around back of other ankle, and bend same knee, pulling back.

Hamstring Curl: Resisted (Sitting)

Facing anchor with tubing on ankle, leg straight out, bend knee.

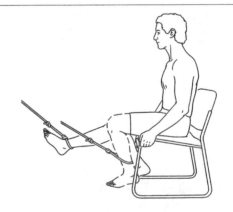

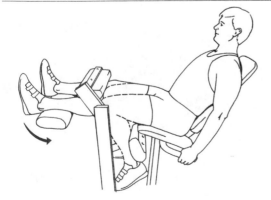

Leg Curl: Sitting (Machine)

Bring heels as close to buttocks as possible keeping feet flexed toward knees.

Leg Curl: Sitting – Single-Leg (Machine)

Bring heel as close to buttock as possible,
keeping foot flexed toward knee.

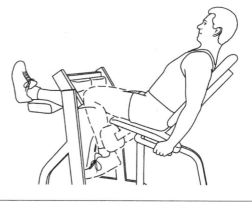

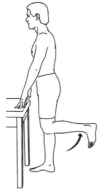

Knee Flexion (Standing): Strengthening

With support, bend left knee
as far as possible. Hold.

Hamstring Curl: Standing (Single-Leg)

In shoulder width stance, anchor tubing under
foot. Loop around other ankle with twist.
Bend same knee, foot toward buttock.

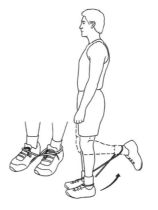

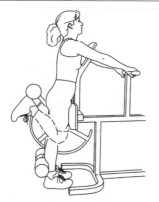

Leg Curl: Standing – Single-Leg (Machine)

Bring heel as close to buttock as possible,
keeping foot flexed toward knee.

Hamstring Curl: Prone (Single-Leg)

Lying on stomach, anchor tubing around one foot. Loop around ankle with twist. Bring heel as close to buttock as possible.

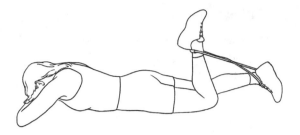

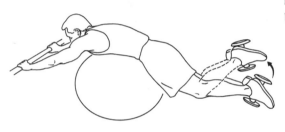

Hamstring Curl: Prone (Dumbbell)

Hold dumbbell between feet and flex knee. Use partner or support if needed.

Leg Curl: Lying (Machine)

Bring heels as close to buttocks as possible, keeping feet flexed toward knees.

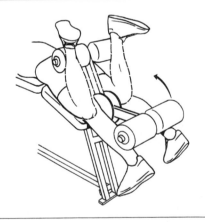

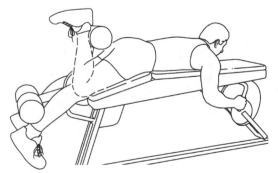

Leg Curl: Lying – Single-Leg (Machine)

Bring heel as close to buttock as possible, keeping foot flexed toward knee.

Leg Curl: Lying (Cable)

Using ankle straps, bring heels as close to buttocks as possible, keeping feet flexed toward knees.

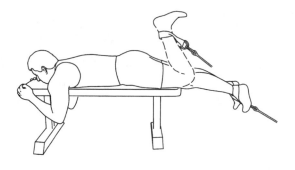

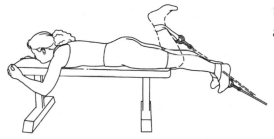

Leg Curl: Lying – Single-Leg (Cable)

Using ankle strap, bring heel as close to buttock as possible, keeping foot flexed toward knee.

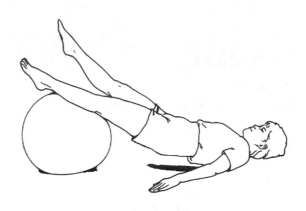

Single-Leg Bridging with Calf on Ball

With calves on ball and hips off floor, raise one leg from ball and hold. Return to starting position and repeat with other leg.

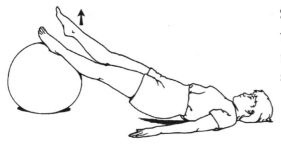

Single-Leg Bridging with Heel on Ball

With heels resting on ball and hips off floor, raise one leg from ball and hold. Return to starting position and repeat with other leg.

Leg Curl with Hips Flat

With hips and knees bent at 90° and heels resting on ball, bend knees so that ball rolls toward you. Return to start.

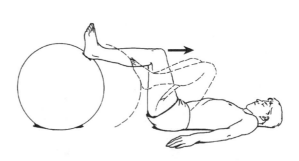

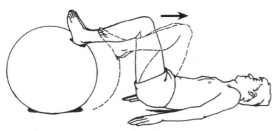

Leg Curl from 2" Bridge

With heels resting on ball and hips lifted 2" from floor, roll ball toward you by bending knees. Return to start.

Leg Curl from 4-6" Bridge

With heels resting on ball and hips lifted
4-6" from floor, roll ball toward you
by bending knees. Return to start.

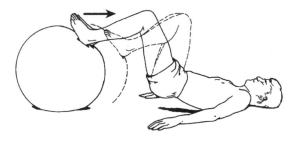

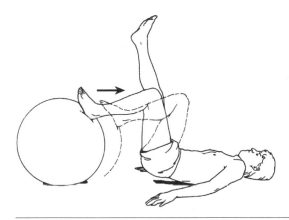

Single-Leg Curl from 4-6" Bridge

With heels resting on ball and hips lifted
4-6" from floor, raise one leg off ball and
roll ball toward you by bending other
knee. Return. Repeat with other leg.

Single-Leg Curl Ball Roll
with Opposite-Knee Extension

Straighten one leg and roll ball toward then away
from you with other leg. Repeat with other leg.

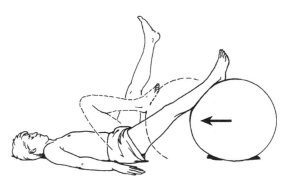

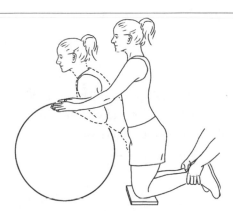

Hamstring Curl: Kneeling

With feet anchored allow body to descend.
Tense hamstrings bringing body back to start.

Dead Lift: Three Quarter (Barbell)

From three quarter squat position, straighten legs, keeping head up and back straight.

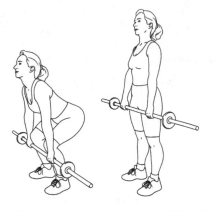

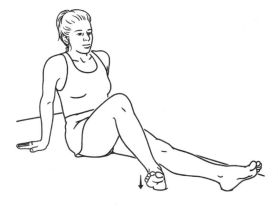

Hamstring Set: Strengthening

With foot turned out, tighten muscles on back of thigh by pulling heel down into surface. Hold.

Hamstring Set: Strengthening

With foot turned in, tighten muscles on back of thigh by pulling heel down into surface. Hold.

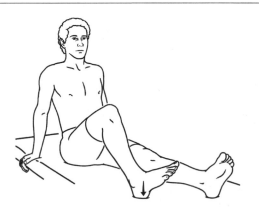

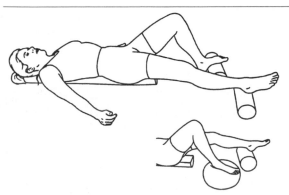

Leg: Roll

Get ON TARGET. Lie on flat up roller, horizontal full roller under each foot. Bend and straighten alternate legs. Check body alignment frequently.

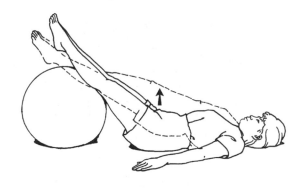

Hip Extension Bridging
with Calves on Ball

With calves resting on ball, lift hips off floor and return. Keep knees straight.

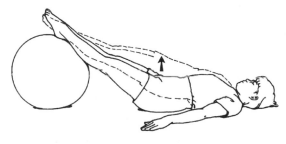

Hip Extension Bridging with Heels on Ball

With heels resting on ball, lift hips off floor and return. Keep knees straight.

Hip Extension Bridging
with Heels on Ball: Slow March

With heels resting on ball and hips off floor, slowly raise one leg 4-6" from ball. Repeat with other leg and perform in a rhythmic fashion. Keep knees straight.

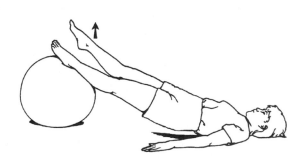

Chapter 4: Gluteals

The Gluteals are three muscles on the posterior pelvis that insert on the proximal femur. The more superficial one - gluteus maximus (GM) - is the largest muscle in the body. The arrangement of its fibers make it a powerful hip extensor and external hip rotator. The smaller gluteals, minimus and medius, are hip abductors and medial rotators. These muscles are dealt with in the next chapter. The current chapter has a progression of closed and open chain exercises for the GM but cannot isolate it from the other gluteals.

For the sake of meeting the purposes of this book, we have tried not to repeat too many of the exercises from other chapters when providing exercises for any one part or muscle. The GM presents a special challenge to this effort. Since it is a hip extensor, and is assisted in this role by one of the hamstrings (the biceps femoris), many of the exercises in the Hamstrings chapter apply here. Likewise, since it is the primary hip extensor, any movement that puts the hip in deep flexion and brings it back to extension, especially when the body is loaded axially, will engage the GM. Hence, many of the exercises in Total Leg will use the GM, especially if taken to a hip angle close to perpendicular. Finally, because of its proximity to the lumbar spine and its primary function as a hip extensor, the GM is involved in many movements of the lumbar spine. Thus, almost all the exercises in this chapter would qualify as low back exercises, too.

Gluteal exercises use the following muscles: Gluteus Maximus, Gluteus Minimus, Gluteus Medius.

    Open Chain - 20 exercises
    Closed Chain - 12 exercises

Bent Knee Lift (Prone)

Abdomen and head supported,
bend one knee and slowly raise hip.
Avoid arching low back. Hold.

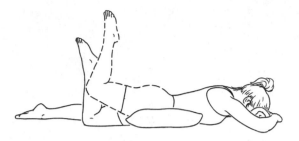

Straight Leg Raise (Prone)

Abdomen and head supported, keep
one knee locked and raise leg at hip.
Avoid arching low back. Hold.

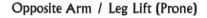

Opposite Arm / Leg Lift (Prone)

Abdomen and head supported, one knee locked,
raise leg and opposite arm from floor. Hold.

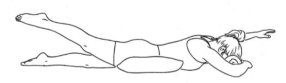

Extension (Prone)

Lift upper body and legs from floor.
Do not arch neck. Hold.

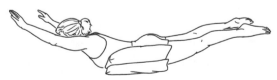

Upper / Lower Extremity Extension (All-Fours)

Tighten stomach and raise one leg and opposite arm. Keep trunk rigid. Hold.

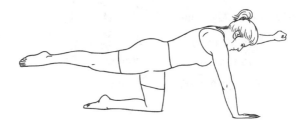

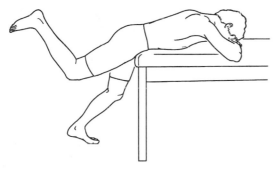

Hip Extension: Unilateral – Support

Leaning torso on table, lift leg, one knee bent. Hold.

Hip Extension: Bilateral – Support

Raise both legs from floor while holding on to table. Hold.

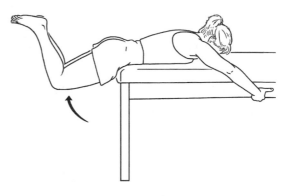

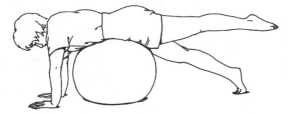

Alternating Leg Raise (Prone)

On hands and toes over ball, raise one leg and return. Do not arch back. Repeat with other leg.

Opposite Arm Leg Raise (Prone)

On hands and toes over ball, raise one arm and opposite leg simultaneously. Do not arch back. Repeat with other limbs.

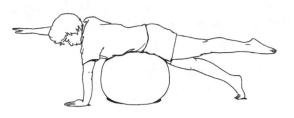

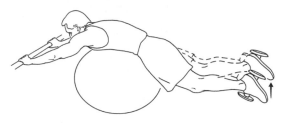

Hip Extension: Prone (Dumbbell)

Holding support, dumbbell between feet, straighten and lift legs.

Hip Extension: Prone (Single-Leg)

Lying over pillow, bolster, or bench and tubing around ankles with twist between, raise leg, keeping knee straight.

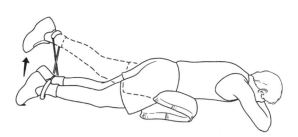

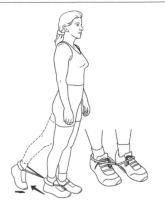

Hip Extension: Standing (Single-Leg)

In shoulder width stance, anchor tubing under one foot. Twist and put around other ankle. Pull same leg back, keeping knee nearly straight.

Dead Lift: Three Quarter (Barbell)

From three quarter squat position, straighten legs, keeping head up and back straight.

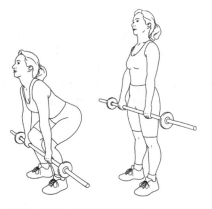

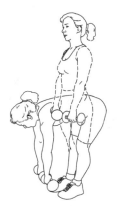

Dead Lift (Dumbbell)

Legs straight, back flat, raise torso until in line with legs.

Dead Lift (Barbell)

From squat, straighten legs, keeping head up and back straight.

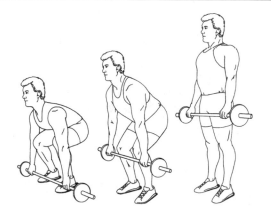

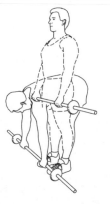

Dead Lift: Straight Leg (Barbell)

Legs straight, back flat, raise torso until in line with legs.

Dead Lift: Twisting (Dumbbell)

Legs straight, back flat, torso twisted, hold dumbbells at outside of one foot. Bring body up, twisting to forward. Alternate sides.

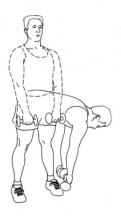

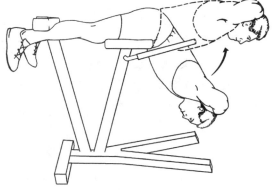

Extension

Bent at hips, back straight, hands behind head, raise torso until in line with legs. Do NOT extend past parallel to floor.

Extension: Incline

Bent at hips, back straight, hands crossed on chest, raise torso until in line with legs.

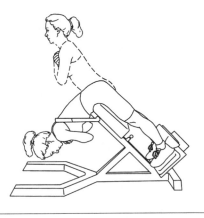

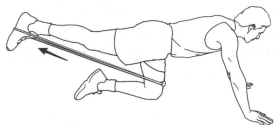

Mule Kick: Hands and Knees (Single-Leg)

On hands and knees, anchor tubing above knee. Loop around other foot and extend same leg back, straightening knee.

Bridging

Slowly raise buttocks from floor, keeping stomach tight.

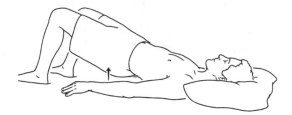

Bridging with Straight Leg Raise

With legs bent, lift buttocks from floor. Then slowly extend one knee, keeping stomach tight. Hold.

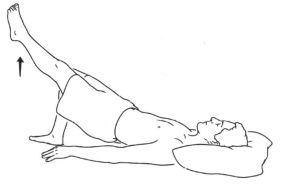

Bridging with Leg Raise

In bridging position with ball under shoulders, raise one bent knee. Maintain balance. Repeat with other leg.

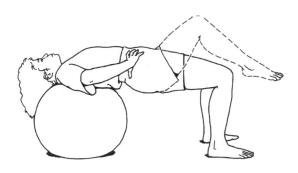

Hip Extension Bridging with Calves on Ball

With calves resting on ball, lift hips off floor and return. Keep knees straight.

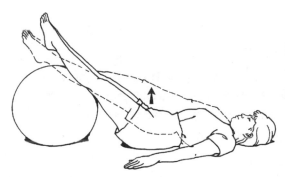

Hip Extension Bridging with Heels on Ball

With heels resting on ball, lift hips off floor and return. Keep knees straight.

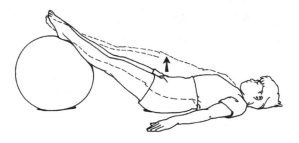

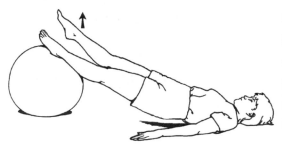

Hip Extension Bridging with Heels on Ball: Slow March

With heels resting on ball and hips off floor, slowly raise one leg 4-6" from ball. Repeat with other leg and perform in a rhythmic fashion. Keep knees straight.

Single-Leg Bridging with Calf on Ball

With calves on ball and hips off floor, raise one leg from ball and hold. Return to starting position and repeat with other leg.

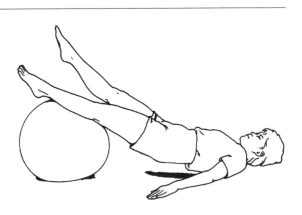

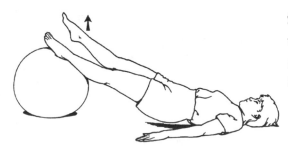

Single-Leg Bridging with Heel on Ball

With heels resting on ball and hips off floor, raise one leg from ball and hold. Return to starting position and repeat with other leg.

Leg Curl with Hips Flat

With hips and knees bent at 90° and heels resting on ball, bend knees so that ball rolls toward you. Return to start.

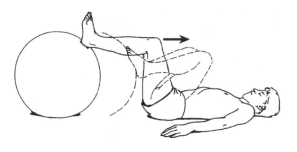

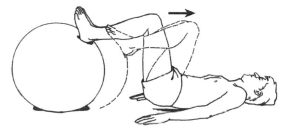

Leg Curl from 2" Bridge

With heels resting on ball and hips lifted 2" from floor, roll ball toward you by bending knees. Return to start.

Leg Curl from 4-6" Bridge

With heels resting on ball and hips lifted 4-6" from floor, Roll ball toward you by bending knees. Return to start.

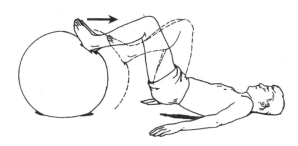

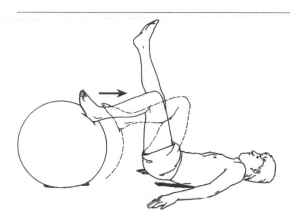

Single-Leg Curl from 4-6" Bridge

With heels resting on ball and hips lifted 4-6" from floor, raise one leg off ball and roll ball toward you by bending other knee. Return. Repeat with other leg.

Chapter 5: Hip Abductors

The Hip Abductors are located on the lateral aspect of the pelvis and femur. They pull the leg away from the midline in open chain movements. In closed chain movements, they bring the pelvis in line with the femur, reducing a lateral pelvic tilt to the same side. The abductors also have a rotational moment at the hip, in most cases laterally rotating the femur. This role has been identified as contributing to proper knee function, especially where patellofemoral mechanics are concerned.

The two primary abductors - the gluteus minimus and gluteus medius - are the strongest of this group; the sartorius and tensor fascia lata (and its tendon, the iliotibial band) are also primarily abductors. The piriformis and the gemelli superior and inferior, also laterally-located hip muscles, are primarily external hip rotators. During gait, these muscles help swing the leg clear of the base leg while the gluteals of the base leg keep the pelvis from dropping to the swing leg side. For this reason, closed chain exercises are deemed instrumental in the proper functioning of the abductors. On the other hand, studies have demonstrated the value of preventing abductor imbalances in the treatment of low back pain, lending value to doing open chain exercises as well.

Hip abductor exercises use the following muscles: Gluteus Minimus, Gluteus Medius, Sartorius, Tensor Fascia Lata, Piriformis.

Open Chain - 12 exercises
Closed Chain - 6 exercises

Hip Abduction – Isometric: Strengthening

Using ball or folded pillow, push outside of knee into wall. Hold.

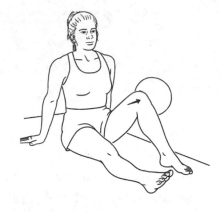

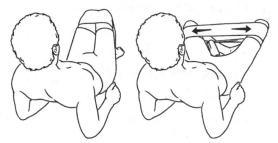

Hip Abductor – Resisted: Strengthening

With band looped around both legs above knees, push thighs apart. Return slowly.

Hip Abduction: Modified

Lying on side with pillow between thighs, raise top leg from pillow, rotating slightly out.

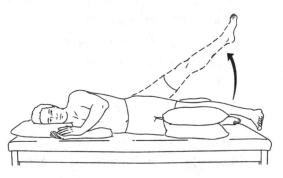

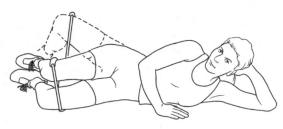

Hip Abduction: Side-Lying (Single-Leg)

Lie on side with knees bent, tubing around thighs just above knees. Raise top leg, keeping knee bent.

Hip Abduction: Side-Lying (Single-Leg)

Side-lying, tubing around ankles, raise top leg, keeping knee straight.

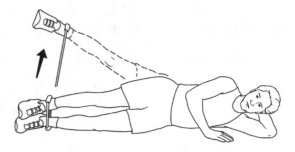

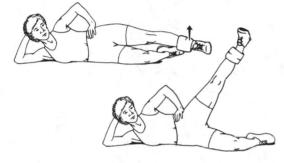

Leg Abduction: Single-Leg (Ankle Weight)

Top leg weighted and straight, sweep leg upward as far as possible. Complete all repetitions to one side. Repeat on other side.

Hip Abduction: Standing - Straight Leg

In shoulder width stance, tubing around ankles, pull leg out to side, keeping knee straight.

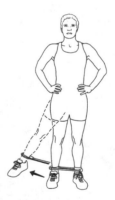

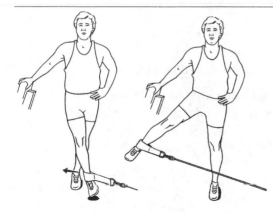

Leg Abduction: Standing (Cable)

Holding support, sweep leg outward away from body.

Leg Abduction: Sitting (Machine)

Move legs outward and slowly return to start.

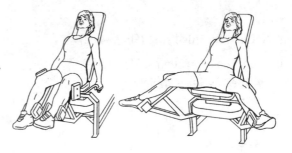

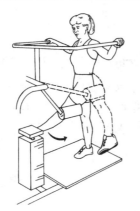

Leg Abduction: Standing (Machine)

Leg across mid line against pad, sweep leg outward as far as possible.

Hip Abduction: Sitting (Cable)

Back straight, knee straight, pull cable out to side.

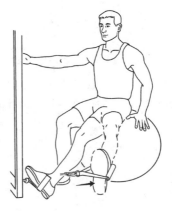

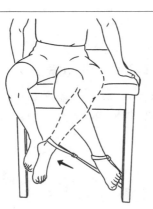

Hip External Rotation: Resisted

Sit with band loop around ankle, anchor on same side. Keeping thigh flat and knee bent at right angle, pull ankle across body.

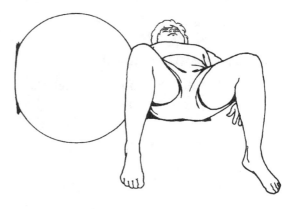

Isometric Abduction in Supine

With ball against wall, press outside of knee into ball.

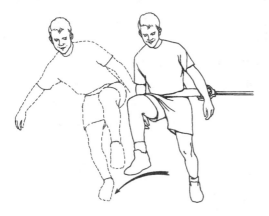

Skier's Jump With Tubing:
Quad Strength, Agility

With tubing around waist, squat to 30-45°. Push off sideways with inside leg and lunge onto the other. Push off with other leg to bounce back.

Rocker Board: Agility, Timing, Proprioception

Standing on board, make medium sliding motion. (May use poles or hand weights.)

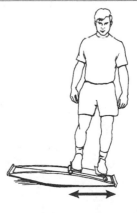

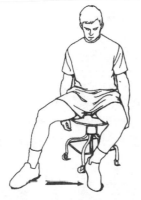

Sideways Stool Walk: Strength, Agility, Timing

Using both legs, "walk" sideways using side steps down a long hall.

Squat Supported: Lateral (Dumbbell)

Back straight, lean into ball. Bend at knee; do not allow knees past toes. Repeat on same side, legs switched. Repeat sequence on other side.

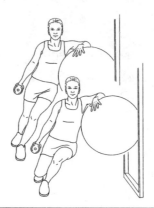

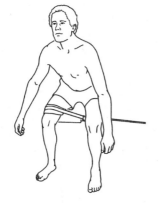

Squat: With Valgus Challenge

Opposite side toward anchor, strap just above knee of leg, squat by dropping hips as if sitting in chair. Do not allow strap to pull knee in.

Chapter 6: Hip Adductors

The Hip Adductors pull the thigh toward the midline of the body and, when the foot is on the ground, the pelvis more completely over the base leg and foot. The balanced forces of the adductors and abductors maintain the proper alignment of the pelvis over the knee and ankle. If one is pulling harder, or is weaker than the other, pelvic alignment may create problems along the kinetic chain superiorly, in the spine, or inferiorly, at the knee and maybe the ankle. Like the abductors, their actions vary according to whether they are acting on an open-chain limb or a closed-chain limb. For that reason, exercises of both sorts are recommended.

The adductors are four muscles that originate at the hip to bring the femur to the midline: the adductor longus, adductor brevis, adductor magnus, and the gracilis. These four muscles insert on the medial aspect of the femur such that their direction of pull is directly in the frontal plane. They may have some role in hip flexion. Some of the fibers have a medial rotational pull on the femur; some fibers attached posterior to the femur's medial edge may help in lateral rotation. The controversy about their role in rotation is further compounded by the position of the femur when they contract. If medially rotated, they exert a more medial rotation torque. If the femur is laterally rotated, the fibers align to have a more lateral rotation torque. The adductors longus and magnus have fibers that intertwine with the vastus medialis and are believed useful in training the vastus medialis for better patella control. The gracilis helps stabilize the knee medially, and may assist in medial rotation at the knee.

The Hip Adductor exercises use most if not all of the following muscles: Adductor Longus, Adductor Magnus, Adductor Minimus, Adductor Brevis and Gracilis.

Open Chain - 11 exercises
Closed Chain - 3 exercise

Hip Adduction: Isometric Strengthening

With ball or folded pillow between knees, squeeze knees together. Hold.

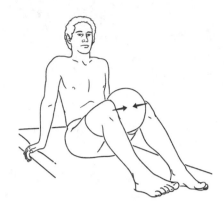

Isometric Adduction in Supine

Lying flat on back, squeeze ball between knees.

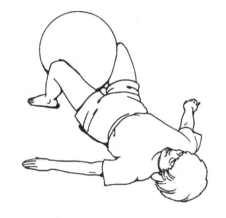

Hip Adduction: Single-Leg Strengthening

Tighten muscles on front of right thigh, then lift leg from surface, keeping knee locked.

Hip Adduction: Single-Leg (Tubing)

Side-lying, anchor tubing under foot of bent leg. Loop around ankle of straight leg with twist. Raise bottom leg, keeping knee straight.

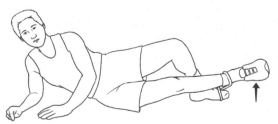

Leg Adduction: Single-Leg
(Ankle Weight)

Bottom leg weighted and straight, lift leg upward as far as possible. Complete all repetitions to one side. Repeat on other side.

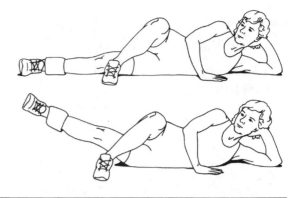

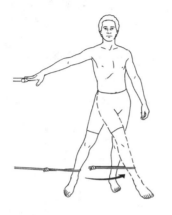

Hip Adduction: Resisted Strengthening

With tubing around leg nearest anchor, bring leg across body.

Leg Adduction: Standing (Cable)

Holding support, sweep leg inward across body.

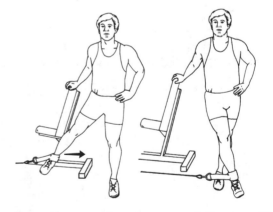

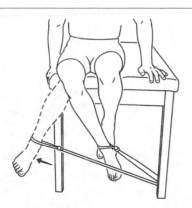

Hip Internal Rotation: Resisted

Sit with band loop around ankle, anchor on other side. Keeping thigh flat and knee bent at right angle, pull ankle away from body.

Leg Adduction: Sitting (Machine)

Legs separated, move legs together
and slowly return to start.

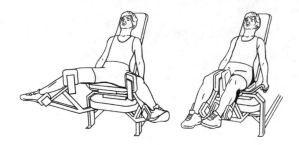

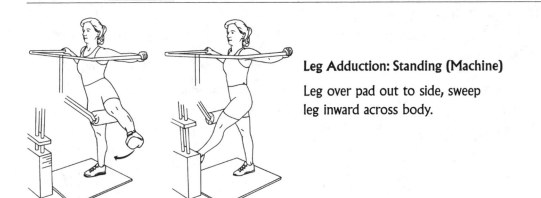

Leg Adduction: Standing (Machine)

Leg over pad out to side, sweep
leg inward across body.

Cross-Over Step With Tubing: Timing, Agility

With tubing around waist, cross over foot of involved leg. Return.

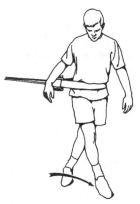

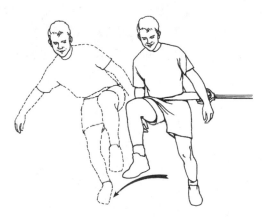

Skier's Jump With Tubing: Quad Strength, Agility

With tubing around waist, squat to 30-45°. Push off sideways with inside leg and lunge onto the other. Push off with other leg to bounce back.

Squat Supported: Lateral (Dumbbell)

Back straight, lean into ball. Bend at knee; do not allow knees past toes. Repeat on same side, legs switched. Repeat sequence on other side.

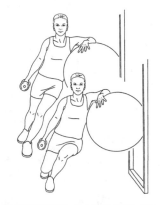

Chapter 7: Lower Leg Muscles

The muscles of the Lower Leg primarily control the ankle. The ankle dorsiflexes (toes lift toward the shin), plantar flexes (toes point), inverts (supinates), and everts (pronates). These movements help the foot avoid hitting the ground as you bring the leg forward during gait, and enable it to both absorb the shock of landing and propel the body forward in push-off.

The posterior muscles that plantar flex are the gastrocnemius and soleus, operating with a single tendon, the Achilles tendon. The former is a two joint muscle that helps flex the knee, too. It has two heads, the lateral and medial, and can be trained in some measure of isolation by the rotation of the hip medially and laterally, respectively. The soleus, on the other hand, only works at the ankle. Both plantar flex the ankle but the gastrocnemius will have a compromised force production when the knee is flexed. These two muscles are often referred to as the triceps surae.

The anterior shin muscle - the tibialis anterior - dorsiflexes the ankle. It also inverts the foot. This muscle's strength relative to the triceps surae may be a factor in the treatment and prevention of "shin splints". The peroneal muscles, brevis and longus, lie on the lateral lower leg. They evert the foot and assist in plantar flexion. They are important in providing active stabilization of the ankle against inversion injuries.

Lower Leg exercises use one or more of the following muscles: Triceps Surae (Gastrocnemius and Soleus), Tibialis Anterior, Peroneus Longus, and Peroneus Brevis.

> Gastrocnemius & Soleus:
> > Open Chain - 5 exercises
> > Closed Chain - 12 exercises
> > Machines - 5 exercises
> Tibialis Anterior - 5 exercises

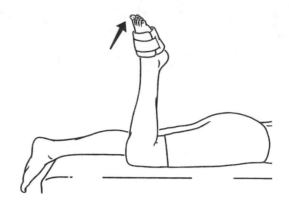

PRE: Plantar Flexion – Knee Flexed (Prone)

Lying on stomach with knee bent and weight around foot, point foot toward ceiling.

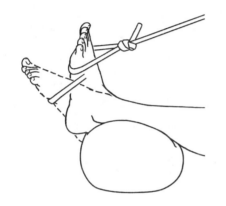

Plantar Flexion: Resisted

Anchor behind, tubing around foot, press down.

PRE: Eversion (Side-Lying)

With weight around foot, big toe down, bend ankle up and turn foot out.

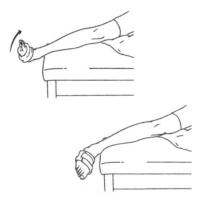

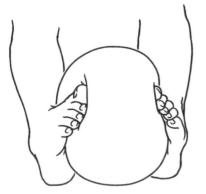

Inversion: Isometric

Press inner borders of feet into ball or rolled pillow between feet. Hold. Relax.

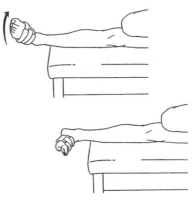

PRE: Inversion (Side-Lying)

With weight around foot, big toe up,
bend ankle up and turn foot in.

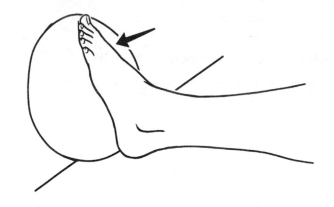

Plantar Flexion: Isometric

Press foot into ball or rolled pillow against wall. Hold. Relax.

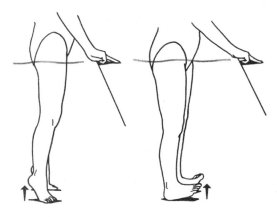

Toe / Heel Raise

Gently rock back on heels and raise toes. Then rock forward on toes and raise heels.

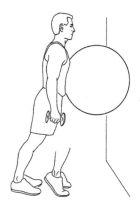

Calf Raise Supported (Dumbbell)

Lean on ball and rise up onto toes.

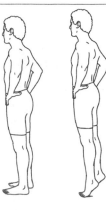

Heel Raise: Bilateral (Standing)

Rise on balls of feet.

Heel Raise: Unilateral (Standing)

Balance on one foot, then rise on ball of foot.

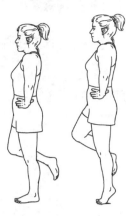

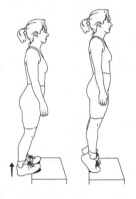

Heel Raise: Standing

Toes on board, heels on floor, knees slightly bent, rise up on toes as high as possible.

Heel Raise: Standing (Dumbbell)

Toes on board, heels on floor, knees slightly bent, rise up on toes as high as possible.

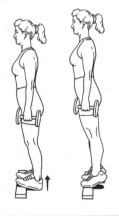

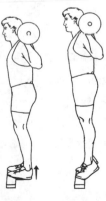

Heel Raise: Standing (Barbell)

Toes on board, heels on floor, knees slightly bent, rise up on toes as high as possible.

Heel Raise (Sitting)

Raise heels, keeping toes on floor.

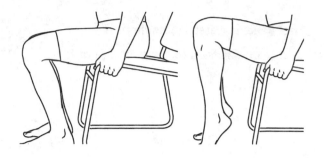

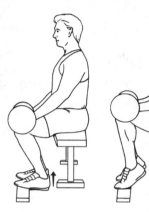

Heel Raise: Sitting (Barbell)

Toes on board, heels on floor, and barbell on lower thighs, rise up on toes as high as possible.

Calf Raise: Sitting (Dumbbell)

Rest dumbbells on thighs and rise up on toes.

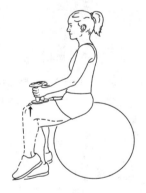

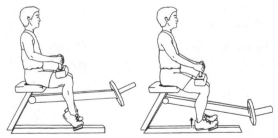

Heel Raise: Sitting (Machine)

Weight on lower thighs, rise up on toes as high as possible.

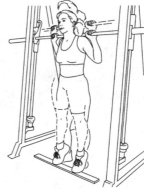

Heel Raise: Standing (Smith Machine)

Toes on board, heels on floor, knees slightly bent, rise up on toes as high as possible.

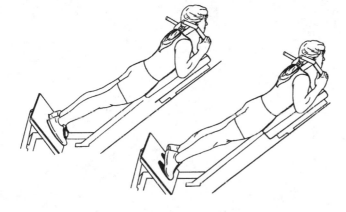

Hack Squat Heel Raise

From starting position, facing machine, rise up on toes as high as possible.

Heel Raise (Machine)

Legs extended, knees slightly bent, rise up on toes as high as possible.

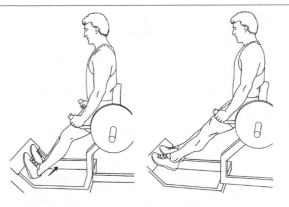

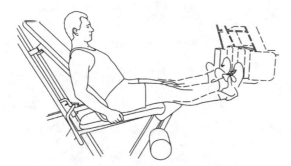

Heel Raise: Sitting (Machine)

Ankles flexed and calves stretched, press toes forward as far as possible.

Heel Raise – Incline (Machine)

Ankles flexed and calves stretched, press
toes forward as far as possible.

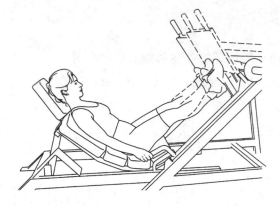

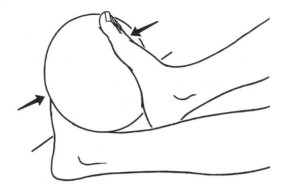

Dorsiflexion: Isometric

With ball or rolled pillow between feet, squeeze feet together. Hold. Relax.

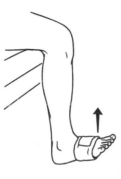

PRE: Dorsiflexion

Sitting with leg over edge of table or bed and weight around foot, flex ankle, moving toes toward knee.

Dorsiflexion: Resisted

Facing anchor, tubing around foot, pull toward face.

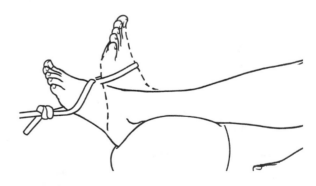

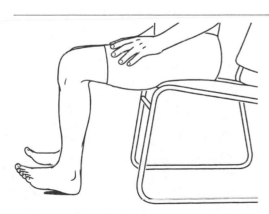

Toe Raise (Sitting)

Raise toes, keeping heels on floor.

Toe Raise (Standing)

Rock back on heels.

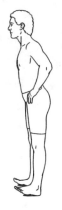

About VHI

Visual Health Information (VHI) is the leading publisher of reproducible exercise tools. VHI has been producing exercise collections for the rehabilitation and fitness markets since 1980.

VHI produces reproducible exercise cards and computer software. VHI has over 35 different exercise collections. These collections include exercises for Outpatient Physical Therapy, Geriatrics, Pediatrics, Fitness, Strength & Conditioning, Pre/Postnatal, Speech, Pulmonary Rehab and much more.

The content for the Exercise Idea book series is derived from the over 9,000 exercise images in the VHI exercise database. These books are designed to show you the wide range of exercises that can be used for specific purposes.

To view all the VHI offerings and collections, visit **www.vhikits.com,** or call **1-800-356-0709.**